The Health Literacy Guide to Stress: The Good, the Bad, the Ugly

Contents

Introduction

Welcome to my third Health Literacy Guide. In this one we are going to tackle a health problem that impacts 100% of Americans at one point or another...Stress.

If you have read the first or second guide, you know I take these books right from classes I have been teaching for the last five years or so. These classes are based on the concepts involved in Health Literacy—the ability to navigate the health care system in sickness and in health and to make good daily choices in your life based on your particular health concerns and how to respond in a public health emergency. Stress is one of the key home problems that often leads people to use and abuse our health care system. Reducing stress leads to healthier lives overall.

Stress is such a serious concern that the Occupational Safety and Health Association (OSHA) has declared it a workplace health hazard. Stress lowers our immune system, ups our blood pressure, eats into our mental stability, makes interactions with the world around us harder, and can make us feel so uncomfortable it can eat away at our spiritual health as well. We need to be able to find good ways to lower our stress and live in health and wellness.

The first three chapters in this book are very similar to the first three in the rest of the Health Literacy Guides because the books are designed to be read in any order, but you need the basic understanding of Public Health, Health Literacy, and Health in general in order to get the most out of the rest of the book.

I hope this book gives you a better idea of what stress is and how to make it work for you instead of against you.

Thanks to William for letting me share his story with you all. And to Alyssa Plock who continues to be the person who reduces my stress as I write these books.

Karen Laing

Chapter 1: What is Public Health?

"Good Afternoon, My name is Karen Laing and I am a public health educator. Does anyone know what public health is?" I use this opening line in every class I teach. Unless I am teaching in a community that hires me regularly, I am usually met by blank stares and a lot of head shaking. And why would you know what public health is? It is the hidden side of the medical system. The prevention piece of the US Healthcare system which works well for some, not at all for a few, and okay for most. Public health studies death, dying, and illnesses to help Americans to live as long as possible with minimum disability.

Public health has five areas of sub-specialties. The first is the research division, also known as epidemiology. These researchers are often found in state and federal health departments and they are the people who put out the contradictory test results, like coffee is good for you, coffee is bad for you, coffee is good for you. At this moment, research shows the drink one makes from coffee beans is good for you…as long as you don't smoke cigarettes with it, dunk donuts into it, or put tons of cream and sugar into it, and if your body can handle the caffeine that naturally occurs within the coffee bean.

The coffee research is a great example of why research is often contradictory and further studies often need to be done. Public health research does not want to assume anything: it needs to prove that the core issue and not anything else is responsible for the results. So when coffee was first deemed bad for you, there hadn't been a close look at the research taking out the effects having a cigarette with your coffee. Cigarettes have been proven over and over again to be horrible little sticks of destruction, and once the results separated out the coffee-only addicts vs the coffee-and-cigarette addict, coffee seemed healthier. When studies separated out those who drank coffee but paired it with highly un-nutritious food (like donuts and desserts), coffee again improved in the health realm. And again there was a difference between those who drank their coffee black, those who only used a little flavoring, and those who liked "a little coffee with their cream and sugar." Then finally, research goes to an individual level. Some of the most recent reports are showing extremely positive results from drinking coffee like less depression, long-term memory, less sin cancer, liver disease and gout. Then of course there is the question, How did your body process the caffeine? If you can't handle caffeine, then coffee might be just fine for your neighbor and no good for you. Just like strawberries are great, unless you are allergic to them, then you should not eat them.

Once the statisticians in the research field are pretty sure they can link a cause and effect together, they will often send the research to the second division- public policy. This is where that research goes to creating laws to keep us safe. Fluoride in drinking water, and seat belt laws are two of the US's most well-known public health policies or laws.

The environmental health section, the third division, made a huge impact in the clean air and water acts from the 60s and 70s as well as more recently with fracking and Legionnaire's disease prevention. While I was editing the first book, Hurricane Harvey hit Houston. Houston is a city known for very few grassy areas (green space as it is called in public health.) Environmental health was already aware that the more green space there is, the healthier residents and employees tended to be. Perhaps because nature has a calming effect on people, perhaps because there is extra oxygen in the atmosphere from the plants. Now, with no green space in Houston, there is nowhere for the water to go to. Estimates are it could be as long as two months before the water recedes/evaporates. I am sure the environmental public health division will be closely studying the effects on the buildings and people's health when the water floods a building and city for two months in comparison to the areas around Houston that had the same intensive rain, but had green space for the water to be absorbed into the ground. Look for public policy to start changing laws about the amount of green space needed for building in a year or so (the end of 2018.)

Biotechnology is the fourth subdivision. Current technology is studied and continuously improved upon. Oxygen tanks that were highly combustible, heavy, and very limiting to how far a senior could go with it have been replaced with oxygen concentrators that are lighter weight, have little risk of exploding and simply need to be plugged in to work. The lighter weight equipment combined with the increased safety has seriously improved the daily lives of those who need extra oxygen to live. Again, one can see the public health focus toward allowing people to live as full a life as possible despite the chronic illness they live with.

Finally, I come to the last specialty area—social, behavioral and community health. How does public health change a large society to live healthier lives? One of the ways public health does this is through vaccine clinics in stores that make it convenient for people to be vaccinated. Or through public health educators who run trainings to help people understand their illnesses better. Since I started this book with the comment, I am a public health educator; you can see that this is my specialty. I train, less on specific diseases, but on a set of core values called "Health Literacy."

Chapter 2: What is Health Literacy?

According to the US government health literacy is "the degree to which individuals have the capacity to obtain, process, and understand basic health information and services needed to make appropriate health decisions." In other words, it is a core set of skills YOU need to navigate the healthcare system (in sickness and in health), make healthy decisions at home, and (I have included) respond in a public health emergency. Health Literacy is understanding the ABCs of the healthcare system. Most public health educators teach on specific diseases, I teach on skills and knowledge that underlie those diseases.

Health literacy, like financial literacy, is a concept we are just beginning to recognize as key to a successful long life. If you don't know the basics of balancing a checkbook, you are inevitably going to bounce some checks along the way. If you don't understand the how and whys of taking medications (for example), you will make mistakes and end up potentially harming yourself or others.

In the United States, it is estimated that only 1 out of 10 Americans is proficient in health literacy skills. And when the mental health system is involved, the numbers go down to 1 out of 33 patients. The US medical system first recognized that patients were not fully health literate in the 1980s. Back then AIDS patients and Breast Cancer Patients both began demanding the right to be involved in their own care. They wanted to make decisions about treatment and lifestyle choices and when to end treatment. As doctors handed patients over the right to make decisions, they realized that not all patients could make the right decisions. Medical schools responded to low health literacy by teaching doctors to use "plain language," translators, and to provide education guides with pictures. While this was a good step toward better communication, it did not solve a patient's ability to ask questions and feel competent to make decisions. It changed the doctor's way of communicating, but did not improve the health literacy skills of the patients.

In 2012, I found myself studying health literacy for a college internship. I was asked to design a tool to help a poverty-based agency screen which of its clients needed training in health literacy. It did not take long to realize that since only 1 in 10 people were health literate, the answer was not to screen, but to train everyone. I then researched what was available to train on health literacy skills. Since it was 20 plus years since the US had identified the problem, I thought it would be easy to put together some trainings for the everyday patient to use. Sadly, that was not the case. The public health sector was still fighting over whether health literacy included skills or knowledge, as well as how to assess patients' abilities to navigate. As a retail trainer for years and a special education teacher to start my career, it made more sense to me to start training people and see how that improved health literacy skills. And so I created the first health literacy training program in the country designed to teach everyone on these basic skills. I used the bits of curriculum I could find from cancer, heart disease, and diabetes education, along with my training as a researcher to read through the latest research. I wanted to find the pieces of knowledge and define the communication aspects that would help patients clearly share with their doctors about their health concerns, needs, and values.

When I started my work, only California taught directly to patients, and they taught only to low income parents who used Medicaid. By the time I was done with my internship, Florida had also developed a program under its English as a Second Language program. A year later, Minnesota began teaching to seniors. To the best of my knowledge, we are the only four programs focused on teaching skills directly to patients anywhere in the world even now 5 years after I started researching this. The rest of the country and the world are still trying to correct a patient deficit by retraining medical providers. In 2016, the agency I helped open won an Award from the New York State Public Health Association for Outstanding Leadership in Public Health for our work as Health Literacy advocates and trainers.

So why is it crucial that people have good health literacy skills? According to the federal report Inadequate Health Literacy A Barrier to Patient Care, patients who do not have good skills struggle unnecessarily and at a high cost. They are

1. More likely to report poor health status
2. Twice as likely to be hospitalized
3. Remain in the hospital more days per each admission
4. Have 1 more outpatient visit per year
5. Have more difficulty using metered inhalers

6.   Have worse HbA1c levels (blood sugar levels)
7.   More likely to make medication errors
8.   Less likely to comply with recommended treatments.

As a result, they are more likely to be seriously disabled or die at an earlier age than someone with excellent health literacy skills. According to the National Action Plan to Improve Health Literacy, lack of health literacy skills costs the United State between $106 and $236 billion annually in medical bills alone, and an additional $238 billion in wasted medications. As you can see, it is important that public health get to the hard work of teaching Americans to improve their health literacy skills to help control medical expenses as we simultaneously help people live longer.

Chapter 3: What is Health?

Within the first few minutes of every presentation, I like to ask the questions, "What do you think health is?" and "Are you healthy?" Most people answer the first question with comments like, being able to do what you want, getting out of bed in a good mood, exercise, eating fruits and vegetables. In other words we tend to think of health as a primarily physical thing with a bit of a mental health piece to it. But according to the World Health Organization, health consists of physical, mental, social and spiritual health. It is important that we look closely at all four aspects of health.

Most people have a pretty good idea of what physical health encompasses. Physical health is why one would see a medical doctor. It includes illnesses and disabilities. Each of us is born with a certain health level and for the rest of our lives, we make decisions to, hopefully help us stay that healthy or even get healthier. Exercise, enough sleep, good nutrition, avoiding bad habits, and learning to reduce stress are all included in the decisions made at home that reflect in the medical tests for issues like cholesterol, cancer, blood pressure and blood sugar levels. As seniors, It can becomes harder and harder for them to think of themselves as physically healthy when their physical bodies naturally can do fewer and fewer things.

Most people have a fairly straight forward understanding of mental health, too. Right now, advocates are in a national push to change the term from mental health to behavioral health. Behavioral health includes minor problems like anxiety and grief and a general outlook on life, up to more serious issues like learning disabilities, drug and alcohol addictions, schizophrenia, and Alzheimer's disease. At any time one's mental health can take a serious dive. For some people it can return to normal with a little bit of help, or can lock a person in a world of confusion that is hard to escape. One in four people will have a problem with their mental health at some point in their lives, but not all of the problems are long term, chronic diseases.

Social health is the aspect of health that as Americans, we often think about the least. It includes how we get along with others, as well as how others get along with us. The ability to hold a job, save for the future, make friends, raise a family, and enjoy the world are all aspects of social health. When physical health wanes in our old age, what keeps seniors happy and optimistic is their social health. Seeing their family and friends, living in a community with other seniors who are also socially healthy, having enough when they retire to make their lives easier, all offset the physical limitations of struggling to walk or hear or see as well.

Spiritual health is an area that we, as Americans, often do not discuss at all for fear of insulting others. Spiritual health is where one finds their inner strength to get through the bad moments of life. It is their personal beliefs that help them reach the end of their life feeling that they lead a purposeful life. It forms a core set of values on which people make decisions, including health choices.

Spiritual health and physical health decisions should work together to help people be at peace about what they are doing. No one should put their personal values to the side when making medical decisions. This is one of the crucial areas where health literacy training comes into place. If someone does not want to take a medication or get a blood transfusion because it violates their spiritual values, they need to be able to share that with their doctor in such a way, that the doctor looks for alternative ways to treat that patient.

It's not about ignoring the disease or being non-compliant. It's about balancing all aspects of your health. The same is true of social health. Many seniors will continue treatments past the point they are comfortable with, simply to keep family members happy.

When health literacy skills and all four aspects of health are taught to Americans, it has the potential to really change the way we handle life. Stress impacts all four aspects of health. Which is why is it so crucial that we look at it closely and get the very basics under our belts. Eating healthier improves stress reactions, but if we don't put that together with feeling at peace, how does one make sure they are doing their best for their lives? As Dr. Pete Sulack, a leading expert in stress, says "This is an area where ignorance can kill you." And since public health is all about preventing early death, let's get you out of stress mode and into a long life.

Chapter 4: Stress, the Good

The good news about stress is our bodies need some stress to feel alive and function well. There is an optimum level that everyone has that makes their bodies feel alive and rejuvenated. Thrill seekers need more stress than others. Imagine a rollercoaster. Are you someone that must ride every loop-de-loop coaster? Do you prefer the old rickety wooden ones that rock side to side? Are you absolutely positive you would have a heart attack if you just got in line to get on one? Your answer will tend to give you an idea of how much stress is ideal in your life.

Eustress

The amount of stress between boring and your optimum level is called eustress. When we live within this level of stress, we find joy and fulfillment. You are usually motivated by the challenges of life. Your memory improves along with your immune system responses. Conquering mildly stressful problems are rewarding. Puzzles, brain teasers, playing games, learning a new activity, trying a new exercise routine are all things that create that spark of "can I really do this?"

Chapter 5: Distress, the Bad

The point where we cross our optimum stress point, we pass into distress. Distress moves our bodies into fight or flight mode. It is a great internal resource to have if you are running from a bear but not if you are having an argument with your spouse.

Fight or Flight

Distress triggers adrenaline to be released along with other chemicals in our body creating the fight or flight response. Suddenly our focus sharpens, our vision and hearing come to alert. The dura (the covering around are spinal cord and brain) stretches allowing our nerves to talk to each other faster and our body to twist and bend in positions that may help us avoid the bear's paw when it swings at us. Our heart and lungs work together to get more oxygen to the muscles. The fight or flight response shuts off our digestive system and relies on the food already stored in our muscles and liver. We can run faster, jump higher, lift things we would not be able to lift otherwise. It's designed to be a short term solution to immediate danger and it saves lives every day.

The problem isn't the distress side of the scale either. The chemicals released do prevent us from sleeping well (but then again, would you sleep if you were being chased by a bear), healing our wounds, or thinking clearly. We are operating on instinct—the instinct to live. Nothing else matters in those few minutes. The true problem is when we do not leave the distress side and return to eustress. At that point we move to chronic stress.

Chapter 6: Chronic Stress, the Ugly

Chronic stress is a uniquely human problem. Why? We can think and imagine. We can see all the potential problems and instead of realizing the bear is not chasing us and we can calm down now, we worry if the bear will chase us again.

Zebras

Animals do not have this same ability to worry. Zebras live right on the plains with the lions. They can see the lions all the time. Yet *Zebras Don't Get Ulcers* (a great in-depth book on stress by Robert M. Sapolsky). When they are being chased by the lionesses, their fight and flight system kicks in immediately, but once they are no longer being chased their system returns to stasis (the eustress side of life) in three minutes. Even though the lions continue to be right in front of the zebras, the zebras don't think about the future and they don't fear the lions. We humans think our way into most of our fears and then push our bodies into fight or flight when there is nothing actually to fight or to flee from.

The Cycle of Chronic Stress

Chronic Stress leaves your body in fight or flight mode constantly. What is designed to be a short term solution to avoiding death becomes activated to a consistent in our bodies. Chronic stress can actually trigger a whole host of illnesses and potentially an early death. The chemicals that were designed to stop flooding our body when the danger is gone continue to race through our blood stream making us edgy, depressed, and anxious. The stretching of the dura membrane rubs on the bones and cartilage between our vertebrae (our bones in the spinal column) creating sores and inflammation in our spine. This can add to arthritis, degenerative disc disease and sciatica pain. The shutting down of the digestive system means our bodies do not get the nutrients it needs and over time that convinces our body to store extra fat in case we are starving. This little trick our body has for protection now works against us and we end up overweight or obese.

On top of this, once we have lived in chronic stress for a while, we have a harder and harder time to get out of it. Our anxiety triggered by the hormones that make us more alert now just keep telling our body to release more fight or flight hormones. As our brains stop processing well, we make poorer and poorer choices. We overeat, drink, smoke and behave in ways we might not choose if we could think clearly. Instead of eating healthy foods and exercising and making positive decisions, we "deserve" the junk food or the second, third, or eighth glass of alcohol. We stop sleeping which tells our body there must be danger nearby and more chemicals pump through our body in an effort to save our lives. But our lives are not in danger from an external source, we are now putting our own health at risk. As we don't sleep, our bodies fail to repair minor damage done and this grows to be large areas of internal damage. Autoimmune diseases, diabetes, heart disease all gets worse. All of which leads to more bad choices. Now we feel guilt, frustration, and possibly that we are too stupid or afraid to handle our lives well. We may lose patience with others or ourselves. Now the world around us looks truly terrifying and we send out more hormones reinforcing the cycle of chronic stress.

So how do we break this cycle?

Chapter 7: Physically Healthy ways to Lessen Stress

We break the cycle not by focusing on getting rid of all stress, but by trying to move the distress we feel back to the eustress side of life.

Exercise

Mild exercise is a great place to start. Walking, dancing, muscle relaxation techniques like Pilates or Yoga all help. Try a form of exercise you used to love or a new one. Not a big fan of "exercise?" Challenge yourself to try one new form of movement a week until you find something you like. Google exercise options. Try something odd—archery, fencing, water polo, kick boxing. Are you someone who prefers to work out alone at home, in a group, with one good friend? Do you think having music in the background or do you want silence? When do you want to work out: in the morning, afternoon, or evening? Moving at all for ten minutes a day, three times a day will help to reduce the stress hormones flowing through your body. If you can challenge your body to find the most fun way to workout will naturally turn exercise into a healthy eustress behavior.

Eat Better

Next, work on eating better. Instead of thinking "I deserve this chocolate cake," try "I deserve this apple, salad, or yogurt." Use the eustress side of the scale to turn eating better into a fun game. Get together with friends to try new foods, recipes, spices. Aim for five to seven servings of fruits and veggies each day with no more than one of those serving being juice. Even if you juice yourself, only one serving of juice counts. This is because your body needs the fiber and roughage in the fruits and vegetables, not just the nutrients and vitamins. Some experts are starting to push to seven to nine servings. If you have a fruit or vegetable serving every time you eat, and two at lunch and dinner, you should hit the five to nine servings pretty easily.

Try a favorite fruit or vegetable cooked in different ways—raw, steamed, and roasted are all healthy ways to eat them. Each way of cooking brings out different flavors and textures. Do not assume that because you didn't like it before, you won't like it now. Every seven years, your taste buds completely change. You may have disliked it before, and love it now.

Bigger supermarkets have dieticians who can provide recipes and suggestions. Lots of online recipe websites can show you how to transform a favorite unhealthy recipe into something better. I personally always turn to SparkRecipe.com to start with, they have recipes filed under occasions, by ingredients you want to use, and by avoiding certain things (like low sugar, gluten free, or fat-free.)

Drink Water

Drinking enough water is also crucial. Keeping your body fully hydrated allows your liver and kidneys to clear the hormones out of your body faster. Water allows your brain to function well and make good decisions. For most people 64 ounces of water a day is a good starting goal. Three 20 ounce disposable bottles of water and a glass of juice is a great beginning. Some wellness experts are pushing one half your body weight in ounces of water: for instance if you weigh 120 pounds, you should drink 60 oz., if you weigh 220 pounds, you should be drinking 110 oz of water.

You cannot count coffee, green or black tea, or anything with caffeine in it as a replacement for the water. Caffeine is naturally dehydrating and works against your body having enough water. If you drink a lot of caffeinated drinks, try to cut back slowly on those and increase water. Make charts, graphs, give yourself small prizes for reaching your water and food goals. Again, think of it as a game you are playing with yourself and your body will find it fun and move your hormones from distress to eustress.

Other Physically Healthy Ways

Some of the other things you can do to help you break the cycle physically include conscientiously smiling more, deep breathing exercises, playing music, singing loudly. Getting more sleep, 7 to 8 hours is ideal for many people, will also help you to begin to calm.

Can you think of anything you do that can help move your body from the chronic stress to distress to eustress? Make some notes here or in the borders of the book.

Chapter 8: Mentally Healthy ways to Lessen Stress

Besides physically healthy changes, you also need to focus on doing things that are mentally healthy to reduce stress.

Just this week, researchers released a report that says that business people who see negative moments in business as challenges instead of stress, tend to be more productive and healthier than those who react immediately with overwhelming negative thoughts.

Again, perspective is a key to either staying in eustress or moving to distress. Focusing on what you can control helps this process. My favorite phrase to help me focus on this attitude? "Not my monkeys, not my circus, not my problem." Even where the situation involves "my circus" and some of "my monkeys," there are often monkeys that are not mine running around making it worse. Learning to ignore those monkeys helps me to focus on what I can do.

Positivity Project

If you are stuck in chronic stress, make a list of what is good in your life. If you cannot even do that, ask your friends and family to help you. When I teach this class in a business setting or in a senior housing facility, I will often add a project where everyone writes a brief positive sentence about the other people in the room. At the end of the exercise, everyone has a sheet of paper listing all their best qualities as judged by co-workers or neighbors. I have gotten pictures of these sheets of paper hung up on goal charts, refrigerators, tucked into wallets. This would be a fun activity for a family reunion or at a holiday party. Make sure that every person participating has their name on the top of the page, so they can easily find their paper at the end of the event.

Stop Self-Bullying

I taught this stress reductions class one day to a large group of business people at a networking event. I asked them how many of them had bosses that were bullies (a known work place cause of high stress.) One guy said, "not me, I am the boss." I just looked at him and replied, "When was the last time you told yourself you made a total mess of that presentation, you should get out of this field, or you are really too stupid to do the job." The man turned beet red and replied, "10 minutes before I walked in here. I thought, 'I don't belong here, these people are all smarter and more successful than I am.'" Self-bullying is so very destructive to our minds and it makes it easier to find all the negatives in the world around us, instead of all the positives. When you can see the positives, the negatives look smaller and more like easily conquerable challenges than causes for adding onto your stress and sending you into chronic stress mode.

Attitude of Gratitude

This one might seem obvious, but the more things in your life you can find to be grateful for, the less stress you will have. But it also works to lessen your stress (move from distress to eustress) if you can find something to be grateful for in the midst of the worst moments. One of the people I admire a lot on Facebook is a woman who lost her teaching job a few years ago when her private school closed. She could not find another job teaching immediately and she was challenged at about the same time to do 30 days of gratitude. She found it so uplifting that she is on day 1183 as of Nov 3, 2017. She even did it right through an automobile accident that should have killed her. Instead of posting about the pain and injuries, she continued to find joy and things to be grateful for through the hospitalization and rehab. It's been months, she still cannot put weight down on one leg, she hasn't been able to work, but she is still posting gratitude. It's not about "fake it until you make it" or platitudes like "it gets better with time." She is finding three things every day to be grateful for. What are you grateful for?

Avoid, Alter, Adapt, Accept

Finally, think of it in terms of the Four A's to stress reduction: Avoid, Alter, Adapt, and Accept. The zebras on the plain learn to accept and avoid the lions unless they are in full attack mode. And once the lionesses are done with catching and killing the weak zebra, the rest of the herd adapts quickly to being calm and allowing their bodies to rest. Be a zebra.

Chapter 9: Socially Healthy Ways to Lessen Stress

Our social health also has a lot of impact on our stress in general. Friends can help us find joy and peace in everyday living. Enemies (those who are always telling you how bad it is and how you cannot do better) can be used to motivate you to prove them wrong. The following story came from a friend's Facebook page.

> Seven years ago I got fired from washing dishes because I overreacted to a remark I didn't like. I was given an opportunity to be a per diem Resident Aid at the Altamont program in which I would cover holidays and call outs. I was told that I would never be able to make a career out of this because it did not pay well and I did not have the experience.
>
> Seven years later not only I am the Director but I just recently added a Women's homeless shelter to our program and am working on expanding our transitional groups and abilities.
>
> I am thankful for everyone who believed in me throughout my journey and I am especially thankful for those who didn't. Your lack of belief in me motivated me. To my wife who challenged

me, "You have the opportunity change lives and you are throwing it away," I love and appreciate you.

I am blessed to do what I do and thankful for the struggle that prepared me.

William

Physical Contact

Physical contact often helps as well. Don't forget to ask for a hug if you need one. Find a way to shake someone's hand. Go get a massage. I remember one day sitting in the living kicking my brother's feet and he was kicking back. My oldest son used to need to be wrestled to the ground to calm down. Physical contact in almost any form with another human being can be a calming presence when done in love.

Apologize

Apologize if you did something wrong and verbally accept an apology if someone else apologizes. ("Of course I accept your apology." "Thank you for your apology, I forgive you.") Something about those words brings a level of peace that de-stresses and calms the situation.

Other options

You may want to create a support group if you are dealing with an issue that will not resolve itself easily (like a cancer diagnosis or a boss that is given to temper tantrums). Call a friend. Tell a joke. Arrange a game night. Do something nice for someone else. Mentor. Google Random Acts of Kindness or The Humor Project for some great ideas on how to use kindness and humor to de-stress yourself or others. Remember it's not just you in your world. Stress in your community, often referred to as trauma, impacts some people that may make your stress worse.

Think about the last few natural or man-made disasters. People line up to help. They give blood, build temporary dams, donate money or clothes. We don't want to see others hurting. It is bad for them, but it also increases our stress. So when we reach out to others, we are also self-soothing our stress with the idea that others will be there for us too.

Chapter 10: Spiritually Healthy Ways to Lessen Stress

House of Worship

Spiritually we need to feel connected to a bigger purpose in life to get through highly stressful moments. Going to your church, temple or services is a fabulous way of once a week slowing life down and allowing your faith to help you find peace. Prayer and meditation go right along with that, except those can be 24/7 options. Feel yourself panicking? Pray.

Forgiveness

Forgiveness, mentioned above in the socially healthy ways is also a form of spiritual health. You may need to forgive others, yourself, God, or the circumstances. I love this quote that I read somewhere, "The first to apologize is the bravest. The first to forgive is the strongest. The first to forget is the happiest." We need to both forgive and forget in order to not allow the past to trigger fears that are not helpful in the moment to staying in eustress.

Nature

Get outside and enjoy nature. Nature is there to remind our spirits that we are tied to something bigger than ourselves. When we see ourselves as a small cog in a big wheel, it is so much easier to see our stressors as minor things that can be easily overcome with a little creativity and some time.

For many people gardening or arranging flowers has this same nature connection. Talking to a pet or any animal can help you feel the same way. Caring, even for fish and snakes that might not respond the same way a dog or cat does, can still be a spiritual connection. Dementia patients even do well with the robotic animals that are soft and furry, but also bark or meow. Even a small pillow or blanket designed to feel like fur can be used to calm dementia patients and others who have sensory issues.

God Box It

One of my friends has a small box she keeps next to her bed. When she simply cannot stop worrying about something, she writes it on a piece of paper, puts it in the box, and gives it to God. She admits it took a while before she totally stopped worrying about things in the

God Box, but after several years, she now totally trusts the process. She enjoys opening the box periodically and seeing how God solved that problem. It wasn't always the way she would, but it gives her a deeper faith to know eventually the problem was solved and she didn't have to deal with it. It wasn't her circus or her monkeys after she gave them to God.

How can you connect deeper to your faith in order to lessen the stress in your life?

Chapter 11: Use Your Senses to Relieve Stress

Another way to look at stress reduction is to use your senses to reduce your stress. These are especially helpful in helping you keep your stress on the eustress side of life rather than de-stressing yourself.

Movement

Rhythmic movement, while not really a sense, is a great way to stay calm. Swaying, dancing, fly fishing, drumming, knitting all involve doing something repetitively that helps you slow your breathing, see the positives around you and realize the chemicals in your brain that bring pleasure- dopamine and serotonin. For woman especially brushing their hair (or better yet, having their spouse gently brush their hair) can be extremely calming. Swinging in a hammock or using a rocking chair is also that same kind of rhythmic pattern. Make notes in the margins of other rhythmic patterns you enjoy doing.

Sight

How can you use your sight to relieve stress? Looking at clouds for shapes and animals is a challenge that can be used to move yourself from distress to eustress.

Pictures of nature, family, or a favorite vacation spot are all calming. This is where all the cute kitten and puppy pictures come from on the internet.

Sound

What about sound? Playing music and singing are both options. So is a sound machine with waves, thunderstorms, or babies laughing. Listening to rain on the roof is peaceful for some people.

Watching a TV game show with the bells, whistles, and canned applause can also help. Will you know the answers before the contestants? My dad watched Jeopardy every weeknight while I was growing up. I cannot help when I hear the theme song to feel challenged to play the game and see if I can win. Where you a game show watcher? If not, and you have the Game Show Channel check out some of the old shows, or the new ones like American Ninja Warrior or So You Think You Can Dance? Listening and watching others challenge themselves takes away whatever stress I feel (if for no other reason than at least that's not me falling in the cold water or on the stage!)

Smell and Taste

Smell and Taste often go together. There is nothing better than the taste of a warm cookie you have smelled baking for the last 10 minutes. Comfort foods are named that way because they bring us emotional comfort. You want to make sure you are not overeating them and many times you can find great ways to make them healthier, but sometimes you just need a piece of chocolate melting in your mouth or the bite of a hot wing if you are more motivated by savory tastes than sweet ones. Smells may also be activated by your favorite perfume, a scented candle, or air freshener.

Touch

Touch is the last sense. We have talked about that a lot in the use of hugs, massages, petting animals, and soft blankets. One of my favorite calming rituals is a cup of hot tea. While I appreciate the smell and flavor of the tea, what I enjoy the most is simply holding the hot cup in my hands and watching the steam slowly lift away my cares.

In Conclusion

We have talked a lot about stress here: about the good (eustress), the bad (distress) and the ugly (chronic stress) of dealing with life. Basically, you will never get rid of stress. Your body loves a little bit of it. It's all about controlling the amount you are exposed to it, your thoughts and feelings about it, and your responses. You can choose to see everything in life as a reason to be highly stressed or you can choose to see everything as a challenge to be overcome. Your body loves a challenge, so focus on that.

But also remember that you cannot control people and things around you. I love the beginning of the Serenity Prayer by Reinhold Niebuhr-

> God grant me the serenity
> To accept the things I cannot change;
> The courage to change the things I can;
> And the wisdom to know the difference.

In these four short lines is probably all you need to know to stay on the eustress side of life. But if that doesn't do it for you then try chanting "Not my circus, not my monkeys," or meditate on "Be a zebra."

Additional Books by Karen Laing

All books are available on Amazon.com on either Kindle or in Paperback.

If you are interested in ordering large quantities for your business, church, or organization, you can reach the author at info@healthliteracyforall.org. Put "Large Book Order" in the email. For large discounted quantities please be aware that the shipping time can take 3 weeks. So plan ahead.

Book Titles

Health Literacy Guide Series

Aging with Style

If you are a senior, love a senior, or hope to be a senior someday, this book is for you. We will take a health and wellness look at the hard questions in the aging process... Where will you live? Can you communicate well with your doctor and family? What about driving and senior fraud? These and other topics will be covered. Use this book as a catalyst to having these hard discussions with your family members

Picking Health Insurance

Understanding the basics of health insurance gets more complicated every year. This book is designed to cover what health insurance is, how to use it well, and what are the things you should be looking at when you compare coverages. This book is a basics class so it works whether you are picking from your state's Health Exchange, from your employer, or Medicare. Additional information includes national resources on finding low cost help and understanding a bit about the basics of Medicare

Stress: The Good, the Bad, the Ugly

We all think that stress is "bad" for our health. But did you know that you couldn't survive without some stress in your life. Your body thrives on it! On the other hand, chronic stress can have long term health complications and can make many diseases impossible to successfully treat. Come learn more about how stress impacts health and how to lessen the bad kinds of stress in your life.

Spiritually Able: Help Your Place of Worship Integrate the Disabled with Ease

Every house of worship I have ever been in wants their members to feel like a family and participate fully in the life of the community. It is an integral part of having spiritual health. Yet often we ignore those who have physical, mental, or social health limitations. This book is designed to help your place of worship work alongside other houses of worship to not only care for the needs of the disabled within your community, but get them actively serving too.

The Everyday Christian's Guides to

Prayer

Whether you are new to talking directly to God, you have just run out of things to say, or you feel like no one is listening, this book can help take you from where you are to a closer walk with God.

Spiritual Warfare

We start with the verse, "If God is for you, who can be against you?" and take a closer look at who gets in our way of having a great relationship with God. We also look at what it means to put on "the whole armor of God" as well as the concept of "the weapons of our warfare are not earthly." See how the book of Ephesians takes us on a journey of training for war.

Coming Soon

Health and Healing

God's view of health and healing from a total look at health-physical, mental, social and spiritual.

And as always, if you have gotten something out of our books, we would love you to make a comment on Facebook at Health Literacy for All, on LinkedIn at Karen Burhans Laing, or on Amazon.com by the book. Even better, copy and paste your comment to all 3! Of course the ultimate compliment is to buy another book for a friend!

Be Healthy!

Karen

www.ingramcontent.com/pod-product-compliance
Lightning Source LLC
Chambersburg PA
CBHW060817260726
48660CB00002B/992